FALLING
IS NOT AN OPTION

A WAY TO LIFELONG BALANCE

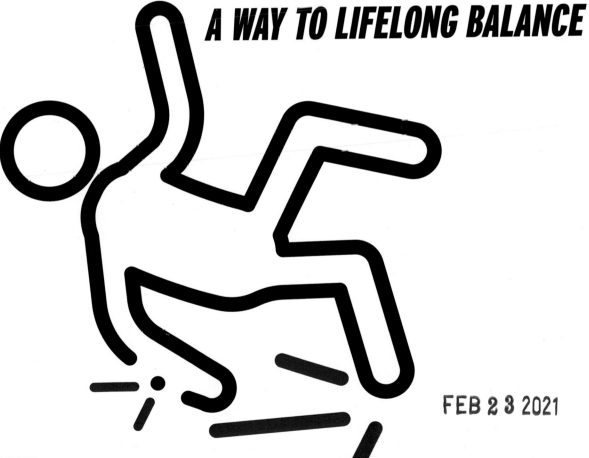

GEORGE LOCKER

Print ISBN: 9781098309732

eBook ISBN: 9781098309749

TABLE OF CONTENTS

DEDICATION

To Chris Molnar, my late wife, who encouraged me to deepen my practice, and whose love and example changed my life forever.

To Elena, my daughter: you rock my world!

APPRECIATION

I have had the good fortune to study Taijiquan and other Chinese martial arts for over 40 years with two masters/teachers. My first, Grand Master Cheng Hsiang Yu, was born in Shanghai in 1929. [1] Master Yu was recognized as one of the foremost martial artists of his time.

When Master Yu moved to New York City, I was his first non-Chinese student *Figure 1*. He spoke no English, and I spoke no Chinese, but he opened a world to me that offered astonishing stability based on a new understanding of the relationship between the body and the ground.

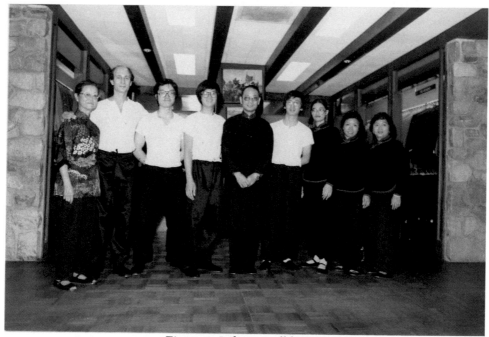

Figure 1: Where it all began.

---

1 http://taichi108.com/masteryu.html

After Master Yu's passing in 2010, I studied with his senior student, Master Robert Murphy, a dedicated and exquisite teacher. Masters Yu and Murphy represent the pinnacle of doing and teaching Chinese martial arts. As would be true for anyone who had two great T'ai Chi teachers and practiced, I am far more stable at age 70 than at age 30.

THANKS

To Arthur Castle, Bruce Esrig, Bob Falvo, Paul Feinberg, Pamela Frank Garry, Michelle Gay, Betsy Jaeger, Nate Jeffery, Mike Sasko, Loretta Thomas, and Randy Young, for their help and support, and to Lester Lefkowitz, for photography.

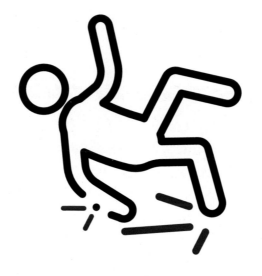

INTRODUCTION

BEAUTIFUL BALANCE

Imagine a child walking along a stream. In some places, the bank is soft and yielding. In other places, there are rocks. The rocks are unreliable: some are firmly seated, and others are ready to tumble.

The child walks on the loose ground, avoiding the moss and sinking into the turf. At a crossing, the child points their toe down the bank, slides, and places their other foot on a rock. The rock wobbles, but the child switches feet again, finding another rock. One step after another, some solid, and some light and uncertain, the child crosses the stream.

This is beautiful balance: the ability to sustain weight while moving in a way that draws admiring attention.

GRACEFUL AGING

As we age, we get drawn into the unnatural world, which does not encourage us to dance across streams. Our agility declines and then must be deliberately restored. What can be done to regain our ability to balance and to enjoy motion?

This book outlines the principles behind beautiful balance and offers exercises* for people of all ages.[2] The exercises are appropriate for seniors who want to improve their balance, mid-lifers who want to prevent balance issues later in life, and athletes who want to take their balance to the next level. In other words, this is a balance book for everyone[3]. Diligent practice over time will help restore, maintain, and improve automatic balance.

These pages contain words and pictures. Ideas and images are important, but experience is essential. In the realm of balance, the body understands before the mind does. Doing the exercises provides insight into the meaning of balance.

To best use this book, choose one location, preferably with a hard floor, maybe a mirror, a wall, and a clear area, practice every day, use a clock, do more than is comfortable, increase the time you hold the postures*, and return to the words and pictures often. Step by step (as the Chinese say), you will cultivate balance and age gracefully.

---

2 Words followed by an * asterisk are defined in the Glossary at the end of the book, in the order of appearance.

3 Mid-Lifers and Athletes see Endnotes.

TEACHING SENIORS

I started to teach T'ai Chi the summer of 2014 in Lake Placid, New York, the site of two winter Olympics. I was hoping to attract future Olympians, but young athletes were interested in any exercise but T'ai Chi. The folks who did show up to my class were seniors looking for ways to improve their balance. Coming from a martial arts background, I wondered how I could relate to older students who had no interest in pushing one another over!

It is said that the best way to learn is to teach. I came to realize that I could offer seniors exercises to improve their balance that were available nowhere else. Their enthusiasm and progress inspired me, and the idea for this book was born.

It took a few years to put into words what I had learned mostly by watching and doing. With help, I came to understand the science and biomechanics underlying T'ai Chi balance and stability. Once I could explain balance in ordinary language, I began to assemble exercises. The postures and movements that follow, which I call Postural Retraining™, are based on my long study of T'ai Chi as a martial art, watching classmates do the same, and teaching balance and stability to older adults.

WHY IS BALANCE A CHALLENGE TO EXPLAIN?

First, while the Chinese have a profound understanding of martial arts balance and stability, the Chinese words themselves only hint at their meaning. For example, the Chinese word for martial arts root includes the ancient character for tree. Knowing this in Chinese - or in English – is interesting but not especially helpful if the goal is acquiring a martial arts root. What does it mean to be like a tree?

Second, there is scant empirical data on how downward force can be increased for the purpose of stability, rather than for creating upward movement. Academic research has focused on large, visible actions, such as running and jumping, to the exclusion of small but powerful movements that lower body mass. We admire the figure skater's beautiful leap, not the bent knee and ankle that preceded it.

Third, textbooks and articles on sports biomechanics don't address how athletes such as surfers or skiers are able to stay upright and stable at high speeds, against powerful forces, often standing on one bent leg. The world of dynamic downward stability is unexamined, so there is little in the literature to draw upon to understand – from the point of view of seniors - how athletes balance and stay upright.

THIS BOOK

We stand erect on two legs. No other creature does. We defy gravity, run, dance, surf the waves. Balance is amazing, but it is hardly understood. What is the capacity we call balance? How does it function? How do we acquire balance, and then lose it? Can lost balance be restored?

The first part of the book discusses what balance is and isn't, how the body achieves balance, how it is maintained, the common reason for losing balance, and why some exercises and sports enhance balance better than others. There is a clear scientific discussion of the physics and biomechanics of balance, which will be useful to primary care physicians and to movement specialists.

The second part of the book presents a unique selection of balance-focused exercises. Each exercise is described in detail and illustrated with consecutive photos of the author holding a posture or doing a movement.

IGNORING THE FUTURE

///

Until it is lost, standing and walking balance is taken for granted, and it goes unnoticed. Although prevention is the only way to avoid imbalance later in life, active adults do not think or talk about their balance. Common imbalance – the condition addressed in this book - does not arise from disease or injury, but from lack of use. [4]

In national surveys, only one in three adults report receiving advice on physical fitness or exercise from their doctor. Racial and ethnic minorities and the elderly receive advice even less often. This is despite the clear understanding that "exercise is medicine" and the ideal time and place to talk about exercise is patient counseling in primary care.[5]

Studies show that when doctors do discuss exercise, it is usually to recommend aerobic exercise, and the focus is cardiovascular. Doctors do not speak to their 40- to 50-year-old patients about balance, which is when the conversation would matter the most.[6] When adults think and talk about their balance, they do so because it has noticeably deteriorated. By that point, seniors are generally inactive and resigned to bad balance. Their doctors have little idea how to help them, so they say to every patient: "Do T'ai Chi." But T'ai Chi is a martial art,[7] and the advice is too little, too late.

---

4 Those with balance issues caused by a medical problem, such as inner ear, Parkinson's, and so on, should try Postural Retraining™ for at least a month and let the results speak for themselves. If balance improves, it is not necessary to understand why or how – just do it!

5 Crump et. el., *Aerobic Fitness and Muscle Strengthening* J Am Board Fam Med. 2019; 32(1): 103-107.

6 https://www.cdc.gov/steadi/

7 For a discussion of T'ai Chi, see end of book.

THE PROBLEM

"Help! I've fallen and can't get up," is an all too familiar refrain. Weakness when standing, insecure balance, and falling are the leading cause of fatal and non-fatal injuries for older Americans.[8] Death from falling is now headline news. From 2000 to 2016, the rate of mortality from falls for those over 75 more than doubled.[9] This is alarming, because common imbalance cannot be treated with drugs or by surgery. It is a medical problem without a medical solution.

It is a belief of Chinese medicine, and it should be obvious to western eyes, that the body ages from the foot up. Balance issues manifest at the end of a life-long process of disuse. Looking around, loss of balance and hesitant walking seem to be—but surely are not—an inevitable condition of aging.

As many if not most men enter their forties, the quadriceps* (thighs) and glutes* (buttocks), which are the two largest muscle groups of the body, visibly atrophy, the legs become spindly, and the ankles and knees become weak and stiff. This spells disaster for balance. At the same time, men often become stronger and wider above the hips, developing a big chest and muscular shoulders. Gradually, walking becomes more difficult because balance cannot be maintained by strong shoulders and weak legs.

As women age, many lose bone density and bone strength. Falls can be calamitous, because the skeleton is brittle. Some balance from the top down, not with muscular shoulders, but with canes and walkers, thereby becoming permanently imbalanced.

---

8 https://www.cdc.gov/HomeandRecreationalSafety/Falls/adultfalls.html

9 https://www.nytimes.com/2019/06/04/health/falls-elderly-prevention-deaths.html?searchResultPosition=1

THE SOLUTION: POSTURAL RETRAINING™

In 1981, along the riverfront in Shanghai, I saw hundreds of seniors doing authentic martial arts-based standing postures and movement exercises. Even though they were elderly, these adults had good balance and they stood securely.

In 2018, in Columbus Park in Manhattan's Chinatown, I saw an eighty-something Chinese woman in a challenging standing posture from a Chinese exercise method called *Zhan Zhuang*, or pole standing.[10] From her steadiness, I could see she had been practicing for many years.

The postures and movements of Postural Retraining™ derive from Chinese martial arts, which developed a deep understanding of balance, stability and movement. Considering that the insights have been tested over hundreds of years, Postural Retraining™ is the ultimate evidence-based balance program.[11]

The weight-bearing* exercises in Postural Retraining™ improve balance in everyday life because they focus on the postural muscles, which are the body's balance muscles. Regardless of age, the potential for improving balance in day to day life is unlimited. Nothing else compares.

---

10 Karel Koskuba 2003; http://www.yiquan.org.uk/art-zz.html.

11 National Council on Aging, https://www.ncoa.org/healthy-aging/falls-prevention/falls-prevention-programs-for-older-adults-2/

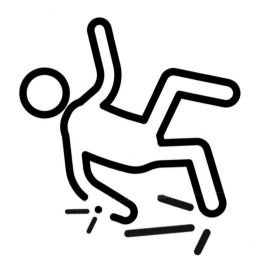

PART ONE:
WHAT IS BALANCE?

STRENGTH?

///

The common explanation for imbalance is weakness, equating balance with strength. This view leads to balance exercises that emphasize building muscle strength.

Balance requires strength, but balance is not strength. Taking a step requires much less strength than sitting down in a chair or standing up. If balance is strength, why do people with enough strength to stand up or sit down, have trouble walking?

Consider balance apart from standing, and consider a young person, not a senior. When learning to ride a two-wheeler, imbalance on a bicycle is not caused by muscle weakness. There are no strength exercises to prepare for balancing on a bike (as opposed to pedaling the bike).

Put a weak young person and a strong young person on a bike (or ice skates, skis, skateboards, snowboards, surfboards, and so on) for the first time, and both strong and weak will fall.

MENTAL?

///

Balance is not mental, and it cannot be willed. In a healthy person, balance is not controlled by the mind. Find a person who can meditate and visualize at a high level, who has never ridden a bike. Show them a person riding and ask them to meditate on riding. Put them on the bike, and they will fall.

SKILL?

Balance is not a skill. It does not require intelligence or athleticism. A complex dance routine can be memorized and practiced, but balance is not attained by aptitude, memory, or repetition.

We can write instructions on how to pedal a bike, because the muscle movements are visible and therefore can be described and copied. We cannot write instructions on how to balance on a bike because the muscle activity associated with balance is internal, not visible, and in any event is not subject to willful control.

SENSE OR ABILITY AT BIRTH?

Balance is not a sense. The phrase 'sense of balance' suggests that balance is sensory. True senses such as sight or hearing are present at birth and function automatically. Balance is not one of the born senses.

Nor is balance a muscular ability present at birth. Large mammals, such as horses, elephants, or giraffes, stand a few hours after birth. An infant learns to stand unassisted only after 10 to 15 months of considerable physical effort.

If balance is not strength, mental, a skill, a sense, or an ability at birth, what is it?

BALANCE IS KNOWLEDGE

///

Balance is muscle knowledge derived from balancing. The body learns balance, not the mind. The child's efforts to stand and walk are the act of learning.

Balancing is something you do in the present in order to have it in the future. My cross-country ski instructor is a senior and a life-long athlete. After he learned standup paddle board, a water sport, he discovered that his balance when snow skiing, which already was excellent, had noticeably improved. Over the summer. he had acquired balance knowledge that carried over into a winter sport.

The body's knowledge of balance is manifested as the ability to stay erect in the face of gravity* and any other destabilizing force, such as a wave or a push. While standing or walking is less difficult than stand up paddle board or cross-country skiing, the body acquires balance and stability in the same way, regardless of the activity.

POSTURAL AND PHASIC MUSCLES

///

The muscle systems of the body belong to one of two categories, the phasic muscles and the postural muscles. [12,13]

The Phasic, or mobilizing muscles, are the volitional*, fast-twitch, movement/action muscles. Volitional means that the mind can direct the phasic muscles to move in a certain way, such as to lift. In an isotonic exercise, muscles contract and change size, and the joints move. Weightlifting* is an example of an isotonic exercise. Most movement exercises are isotonic.

---

12 Vladimir Janda. http://www.jandaapproach.com/the-janda-approach/philosophy/
13 http://wikieducator.org/Postural_Analysis/Postural_and_phasic_muscles

In contrast, the Postural muscles are the non-volitional*, slow-twitch, balance/stabilizing muscles. Non-volitional means, for example, that while the mind can direct the leg to lift, the mind cannot direct the same leg to balance. If the ability is present, balance occurs without direction. If not, it doesn't.

The postural muscles evolved in humans to enable erect standing, walking, and running. These muscles keep the body erect against gravity's downward pull and whatever else is trying to push us down. Postural muscles engage automatically. They do not lengthen or shorten, and there is no joint movement. The work is isometric muscle tension.

As a result of how people today live, work, and play, there is much less standing and walking and a lot more sitting. After years of underuse, the postural muscles literally forget how to maintain balance, even on steady, level surfaces. Falling and hesitant walking is the sign that a lifetime of balance knowledge has been lost.

Because balance cannot be regained by sheer will, this is generally the point when someone who has never thought about balance becomes, or should become, quite concerned because unless addressed, imbalance will take over.

WHY POSTURAL RETRAINING™?

Most balance exercises for seniors address strength and/or agility, which is the phasic muscle system. While exercise of all kinds is good, if an adult loses the ability to balance because of deficiencies within the postural muscle system, balance exercises must address the postural muscles.

Postural Retraining™ is a series of stationary and moving weight-bearing exercises that improve balance because they focus on activating and using the postural muscles.

WEIGHT-BEARING

//

In general, a weight-bearing or weighted* exercise, sport*, or posture is one in which the person is standing, the knees and ankles are bent, and the weight of the body is supported internally, rather than by a straight skeleton. In this body position, the downward pull of gravity can be felt.

Infants learn to stand on bent knees and ankles, constantly falling and getting up. It is this bent knee and ankle weight-bearing position that teach the child's postural muscles to balance.

Cross-country skiing, both classic and skate, and figure skating, are examples of bent knee and ankle weight-bearing sports where body weight is fully transferred from the rear leg to the front leg.

The board sports—wave surfing, snow and skate boarding, and stand up paddle board - are weight-bearing. In each sport, the basic posture incorporates a sustained bent knee and ankle, a lowered body position, body weight dynamically distributed between the bent legs from 0 to 100%. Force is created by rotating (turning) and torqueing (twisting) the upper body and arms, and by rapid downward acceleration. Under this definition, most sports or exercises, even if vigorous, are not weight-bearing.

Walking on an even surface is not weight-bearing. The knee tends to lock when the foot contacts the ground, and the foot does not remain on the ground for more than a moment. Therefore walking, while wonderful and healthy, does not improve balance. (Walking on a rocky Adirondack trail, where both legs are constantly bent to maintain balance, is weight-bearing. Hikers are billy goats!).

Sprinting and jogging are not weight-bearing because the legs, though they are bent, are never in sustained contact with the ground.

Golf and tennis are not weight-bearing, although the rear leg does push powerfully into the ground for a moment.

Unfortunately, most seniors will not or cannot (or should not) take up a weight-bearing sport such as stand up paddle board later in life, even though these sports would offer the greatest benefit to improving balance. Postural Retraining™ provides the balance benefits of a weight-bearing sport without its challenges and risks. The exercises in Postural Retraining™ use the body's own weight to prompt the postural muscles to balance the body.

BENEFITS OF WEIGHT-BEARING EXERCISES

Stimulates the Postural Muscles

No different than a stand-up paddle boarder, the posture that the senior was holding in Chinatown stimulates the postural muscles to balance the body. Dropping body weight* on bent ankles and knees, with a relaxed pelvis and a straight neck and spine, teaches the whole body how to stay balanced. Learning takes place within the entire postural muscle system from toe to head.

Standing with bent knees and ankles is a challenging, whole body exercise. The arms and legs do not move, and it may appear that someone in a Postural Retraining™ posture is doing nothing. The isometric tensing of the postural muscles is internal and not visible.[14] It is something to be experienced.

Sustaining a relaxed weight-bearing posture—not repetition of the posture—enhances the body's capacity to balance. But holding a bent knee and ankle standing posture is challenging. One or two minutes is the limit for most beginners. With practice,

---

14 Rodolfo Margaria, *Biomechanics and Energetics of Muscular Exercise*, Clarendon Press, Oxford, 1976, page 83.

they can be held for several and then many minutes. The improvement to everyday balance will be obvious.

Increases Bone Density

Bone is a living tissue, which changes in response to the forces placed upon it. There is no need to use machines or weights to place a force on the bones. By bending the knees and ankles in Postural Retraining™ and holding the posture, the bones in the feet, legs, and pelvis are stimulated by body weight to produce cells and to become denser.

Relaxation

Weight-bearing exercises are challenging but ultimately simple exercises. There is nothing to memorize or think about. There is no destination except further and longer. What is important is to exercise correctly and consistently.

Warmth

With Postural Retraining™, the postural muscles are working even when in a stationary posture. This increases blood circulation and, hence, warmth. While waiting for a bus in the winter, bend the knees and ankles, hold the posture, and warm up!

BALANCE VS. STABILITY

Balance* is a person standing at rest indoors on a solid, even floor where no force, except gravity, is acting to cause a fall. Stability* is much more than balance. Stability is a person walking on an uneven sidewalk with cracks, or being jostled, and not falling. The goal of Postural Retraining™ is stability, not balance, because in the real-world balance is not enough.

STARTING WITH ISAAC NEWTON

Isaac Newton's insights into physical bodies at rest and in motion provide a basis for understanding stability.

We start with force. Our nerves sense force. When standing, the feet feel the pressure of the ground. We feel the ground reaction force* pushing back at us. It is equal and opposite to our body weight, or downward force*. Newton addressed this opposition of applied force and reaction force in his Third Law*.

When we are not moving and are not being moved, the effect of gravity applied to our mass produces a force that we call body weight. We can't change our mass or weight, but we can decrease the time it takes to move it. This is part of getting good at a sport. It is easier to move our mass down rather than up because gravity is a help on the way down and a hindrance on the way up.

Newton's Second Law* teaches that an increase in the acceleration of a mass yields an increase in force. When standing, it is possible to quickly lower the center of mass* by rapidly closing the ankle, moving the shin over the foot, and bending and lowering the knee. Even a small movement accelerates the body and creates a downward force greater than body weight. This results in a stronger connection to the ground, the surfboard, or the ski. Why is this important?

Faced with a feeling of imbalance, the human instinct is to raise the body. This natural reaction makes the body less stable. When there is a challenge to balance, the stable athlete goes down, not up. By practicing Postural Retraining™, going down can be learned by anyone

ROOTING

As an illustration, put the hands at chest level and press the palms together with equal force. One hand represents the downward force of the body; the other represents the ground reaction force. When pressed together with more force, the hands become more connected to one another. When the two forces decrease, the hands become less connected to one another. The connection exists because the opposing forces exist.

If the downward force increases, the ground reaction force increases, and the foot and the ground become more connected. Being able to keep this connection alive leads to dynamic stability in sport. It is the secret to maintaining lifetime balance.

The horizontal component of the ground reaction force is called the frictional force*. In the example, the greater the frictional force, the harder it is to separate the hands sideways. In the foot/ground situation, the greater the frictional force, the harder it is to separate the foot from its position on the ground—in other words, having a firmer grip on the floor!

The Chinese call the downward force/ground reaction force/frictional force phenomenon the *root**. Inanimate objects can balance, but they cannot root, because an inanimate object (without a motor) cannot accelerate downward. But humans, by means of bio-mechanical movement, can root by generating downward force greater than body weight.

The ground is everything. No matter how strong, we don't leave the ground by swinging the arms up. We leave the ground by pushing the legs *down*. In order to jump, muscle force greater than body weight must be directed *to the foot* to produce upward acceleration.[15]

Rooting is muscle force directed to the foot for the purpose of downward acceleration. The purpose of rooting is stability in place, not leaving the ground. Developing the capacity to root into the ground through Postural Retraining™ translates into improved balance and stability in everyday life.

MOVEMENT IS NOT BALANCE

Experts commonly define balance as the ability to distribute body weight within one's base of support* so as not to fall.[16] This definition confuses movement and balance.

An ability to move body weight within a base of support is a physical technique, the way squinting is a visual technique. Just as squinting is not vision, distributing body weight is not balance. The key to not falling is better balance, not better, quicker, or stronger movements. Indeed, in T'ai Chi, we don't move to achieve balance; first we balance, then we move.

BALANCE IN HUMANS

Human balance is a highly evolved neuromuscular capability. It acts against gravity, is governed by the laws of physics, creates force bio-mechanically, is acquired isometrically, is not subject to conscious control, and is enhanced or diminished depending upon use.

---

15 Chapman, *Biomechanical Analysis of Fundamental Human Movements*, Human Kinetics, Champaign, Il, 2008, page 134.

16 Gonzales, *The Book of Balance*, 60HEALTHandREHAB, LLC, 2008, page 11.

Textbooks on biomechanics relate stability to the size of the base of support. For example, a cone is more stable on its base, than on its point. Thus, an athlete with hands and feet touching the ground is said to have a large base of support, which is presented as being more stable than an athlete standing on one toe, such as a ballerina.[17]

But humans are not inanimate objects. We can create downward force in excess of mass/weight. Is an athlete with two feet and two hands on the ground really in a highly stable position? If so, why don't athletes surf or downhill ski on all fours? Because they cannot generate enough downward force to remain stable.

DON'T SPREAD THE LEGS

Based on the stability of inanimate objects, seniors are taught to spread their legs to increase stability or to stay balanced. As the legs are spread, it becomes impossible to generate downward force in excess of weight, the basis of rooting. It also becomes harder to lift either leg, which limits mobility, making it difficult to move or adjust. In other words, the person is stuck!

When beginner skiers spread their legs, they fall. Expert skiers bend their ankles and knees and push down, usually on one ski at a time. Figure skaters spin the fastest on one bent leg, not on two spread legs. A snowboarder's feet are in a binding and the legs cannot be spread. Where would a skate boarder or wave surfer even put their spread legs? In T'ai Chi practiced as a martial art, stability is achieved on one bent leg, not on two spread legs.

---

17 McGinnis, *Biomechanics of Sport and Exercise*, Human Kinetics, Third Edition, 2013, page 153 and Figure 5.17.

BEND THE KNEES AND ANKLES

A child could never learn to stand up and balance by following any of the available falls-prevention exercise routines. A child learns to stand in a completely different way than seniors are taught to balance.

Surfers in big waves can stand on one bent leg. How is it possible to be more stable on one bent leg than on two arms and two legs, or two legs spread far apart? A wave surfer could never stay upright at speed and high forces if they spread their legs to balance.

A fit adult could do every exercise in every balance book for a lifetime, and never attain a martial arts level of balance. A T'ai Chi master acquires balance and stability in an entirely different way than seniors are taught to balance.

What do children, surfers, and T'ai Chi masters implicitly understand about balance? When it comes to human stability, it's not the size of the base of support that counts. The key to balance and stability in humans is the ability to create downward force in excess of body weight. Thus, neither a statue nor a surfer standing stiff as a statue can remain upright on a surfboard.

How does bending the knee and ankle and pushing into the ground increase stability? The downward force/ground reaction force/frictional force is a dynamic phenomenon that enhances connection with the ground. Unlike spreading the legs, pushing down works!

Note that standing on one straight leg is not the same as standing on one bent leg. When the leg is straight, the skeleton supports the body. Seniors are commonly advised to practice brushing their teeth standing on one leg. There is no mention of bending the knee and ankle of the standing leg, in order to engage the postural muscles.

In Postural Retraining™, the knee and ankle are bent, and the postural muscles learn to support and lower the body and push into the ground, rather than to raise the body. So brush the teeth while standing on one *bent* leg.

WHAT'S THE GOAL?

The goal of Postural Retraining™ is audacious and eminently doable: *zero falls and no fear.*

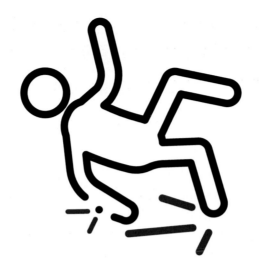

PART TWO: POSTURAL RETRAINING™ ROUTINE

WHERE TO PRACTICE?

//

Indoors on any hard, level surface is fine; a soft rug is not. A wooden dance floor and handrails for support are ideal. Clear away the floor lamps! The back of a sturdy (not folding) chair can be used for balance. Mirrors are helpful. The mind is not a good judge of one's own posture and movement. The eye is accurate, so look. Use a clock to establish a baseline, measure improvement, and to set goals.

It's nice to practice outdoors, but only when there is comfort with the exercises because it's more difficult to stay balanced or to move on an irregular surface. Find a rain-or-shine place and practice every morning.

If dependent on a walker, cane, or even a wheelchair, try to use these items for balance only, not for support. In other words, don't lean on the walker; just lightly touch it. As the postural muscles are strengthened, an external balance aid might become unnecessary. There's no way to know ahead of time.

CLOTHING

//

For freedom of movement and warmth, wear comfortable and loose clothing. Try Chinese cotton-soled shoes, which are available over the internet. Or wear leather-soled dance shoes, or flexible and thin soft-soled shoes. Note that wearing sneakers indoors actually makes balancing more difficult because the foot can't feel the floor and the thick rubber sole "gives." Give the feet a break from sneakers!

WORKING WITH A PARTNER

///

It's helpful to work with a partner who is stable, younger, or who has experience with Postural Retraining™. Such a partner can provide safety, physical support, helpful observations, and encouragement. Of course, two people with balance issues should not partner with one another.

WEIGHT-BEARING POSTURE

///

In Postural Retraining™, the body is slightly lowered by a combination of one or two bent ankles and knees, which is sustained, ideally for minutes. Sustaining a posture is entirely different than repeating a posture. Holding a posture is an isometric exercise that stimulates the postural muscles to balance the body. The longer a posture is held, the greater the knowledge of balance that is acquired by the postural muscles.

When exercising, avoid certain misconceptions: do not think about balance or imbalance; do not try to put the mind in the foot; do not try to feel *chi* "energy." Instead, have no thoughts. Focus on doing the movement or holding the posture correctly. Feel the ground pushing up at the foot. Breathe naturally. Accept a little discomfort as the unavoidable price of progress. As postures are held for more time, everyday balance will improve automatically.

BODY ELEMENTS

///

Foot

In Postural Retraining™, the weight of the standing body is transmitted to the ground through the flattened foot in the area on and just behind the middle of the ball of the foot, slightly toward the heel. In Chinese medicine, the location is called *Yangquan,* or gushing spring. For reference, the internet has many images of this point. *Figure 2.*

Keep the entire sole of the foot on the ground as relaxed as possible. Do not rock back on the heels, twist the foot onto the outside edge, stand over the center of the arch, or stand on, or grab with the toes. Practice standing with a flat foot pushing into the ground on or slightly behind the ball of the foot.

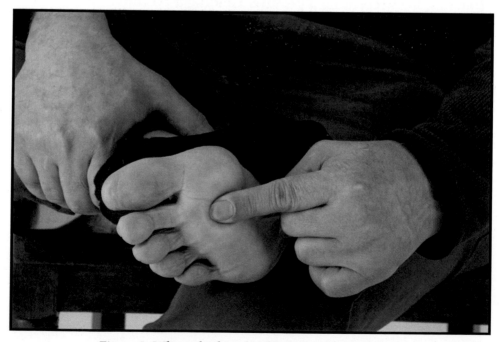

Figure 2: Where the foot should push into the ground.

Ankle

When was the last time anyone thought about their ankle? The ankle is the unsung hero of balance. A flexible ankle allows the shin to move forward over the foot and the knee to bend. If the ankle is frozen, the shin cannot move forward over the foot, and the knee cannot be bent. This is a common limitation that leads to balance issues. There are two ways to close* the ankle in dorsiflexion. Bring the toes and foot up toward the shin, which is limited to 20 degrees at best (Figure 3), or bend the knee to move the shin forward* and over the foot, which allows the ankle to bend far more (Figure 4).

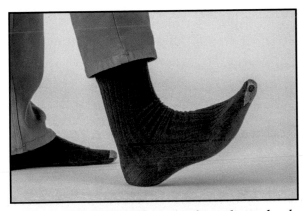

Figure 3: Bending the ankle to the shin is limited at best.

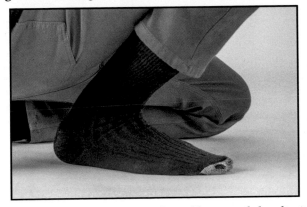

Figure 4: Bending the shin to the ankle is much less limited.

Shin

When standing, if the shin is moved forward over the foot from the heel to the toes, the ankle can be closed* considerably. The knee is bent* by relaxing, rather than by tensing muscles. Relaxing the leg and buttock muscles requires awareness and confidence. Standing up opens the bent or closed ankle*. Bringing the shin to the ankle, rather than bringing the ankle to the shin, is the only effective way to loosen and strengthen a stiff ankle. *Figures 5 & 6.*

For stability and spring, the figure skater closes and then opens* the ankle -dorsiflexion followed by flexion. Being able to bring the shin closer to the front of the foot is crucial to balance and stability in everyday life. With time, Postural Retraining™ exercises will help a stiff ankle to close and open more easily.

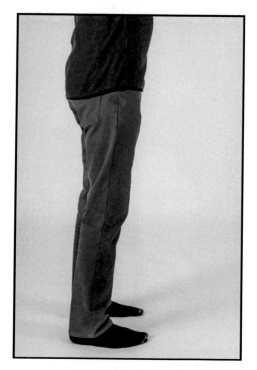 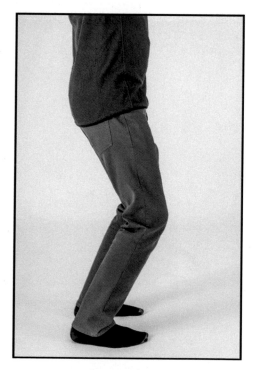

Figure 5: When standing straight, the knee and the shin are over the middle of the foot.   *Figure 6: Bending the ankle moves the shin and knee forward over the foot toward the toes.*

Knee

When standing, keep the knee directly over the ankle, rather than inside or outside the ankle. Some may experience knee discomfort when beginning Postural Retraining™. Stop if there is sharp knee pain. But if the knees or muscles just ache or shake, it is likely because they are being used beyond their usual comfort range. Try not to stop! Tolerating the discomfort of a posture is essential, because the postural muscles need to be activated. With time and practice, the pressure on the knees will be relieved.

Pelvis

Become aware of the pelvis and how it rocks forward and back in its joint. If the lower back muscles are tight and shortened, which is common, the pelvis will be arched back and upward, known as an anterior pelvic tilt.. If the groin muscles are tight, the pelvis may be tilted forward and up, known as the posterior pelvic tilt. For reference, there are many images of the pelvis and its range of movement available on the internet.

The goal when standing is to relax the buttocks and bring the pelvis into a neutral position, tilted neither back nor forward. This will take a while. The squatting exercise described at the end of the book will help to lengthen the muscles of the lower back and allow the pelvis to assume a neutral position.

Spine, Neck and Head

When standing, hold the spine straight but not rigid. The body is relaxed downward from the pelvis, while at the same time it is lengthened upward from the top of the head, like a marionette. The head and neck are directly above, and not forward of the spine. The jaw is relaxed and tilted slightly down. If the jaw is tilted up, the head tilts back and the neck is pinched. If the jaw juts forward, the head and neck will not be directly over the spine. The vertical spine and neck alignment continue upward to the top of the head, to the location known in Chinese medicine as the *baihui*, or hundred meetings. The shoulders and arms are slightly forward of the side of the body, not behind. *Figures 7, 8, 9, & 10.*

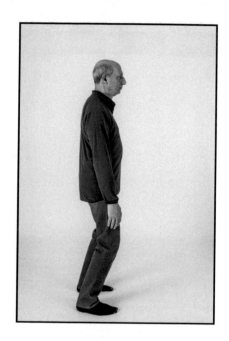

Figure 7: Good posture

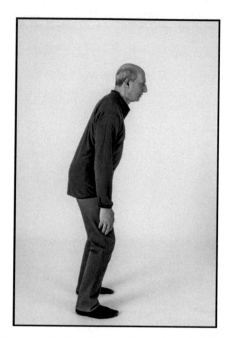

Figure 8: Bad posture - buttocks tilted back

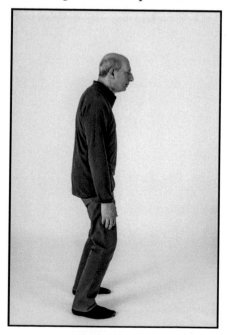

Figure 9: Bad posture - head thrust forward

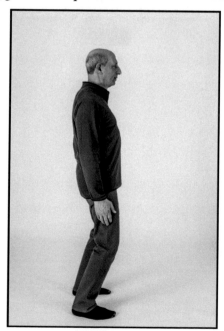

Figure 10: Bad posture - chest thrust forward,

HOW TO STAND

Standing in Postural Retraining™ is different than everyday standing, because the knees and ankles are bent, and the head and spine are erect and vertical. While holding any posture, feel and involve the entire body, from the *gushing spring* by the ball of the foot to the *hundred meetings* on the top of the head.

The bent knees and ankles stimulate the postural muscles to balance, and the erect head and spine mimics their position when standing with straight legs. In this kind of posture, the balancing that is being learned by the postural muscles is standing balance. Whatever progress occurs with these exercises will immediately translate into better balance in daily life, and it will be noticeable.

When the actual weight of the body is supported by both legs, it is called a double-weighted stance or posture. If the actual weight of the body is 100% supported on leg, it is called a single-weighted stance or posture. Postural Retraining™ includes double-weighted and single-weighted exercises, both stationary and moving, to stimulate the postural muscles to balance.

BOTH LEGS STRAIGHT

Stand with legs straight and comfortably spread apart, feet flat on the ground, toes relaxed and pointed straight ahead and on one line, with each foot carrying equal body weight, shoulders relaxed, arms relaxed by the side. The only way to make sure the feet are pointing straight ahead, parallel, and on the same line, is by looking at them.

Each leg holds 50% of body weight distributed through the skeleton. The body's line of gravity* runs down the spine and tailbone and into the floor, midway between the legs.

Locate the gushing spring point by the ball of the foot where it contacts the ground. Notice how it feels when the legs are straight, the knees are not bent, and the skeleton supports body weight. Compare to the next exercise, when the knee and ankle are bent. *Figures 11, 12 & 13.*

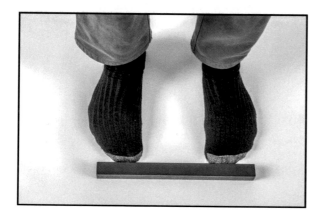

Figure 11: Feet straight, parallel, and even

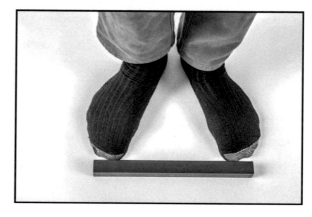

Figure 12: Feet not parallel but 45 degrees

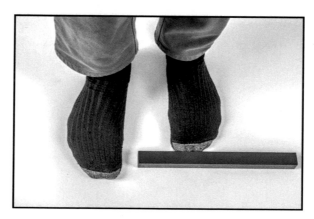

Figure 13: Feet not even

WEIGHTING THE STANCE

Double-Weighted

Stand with straight legs, as above. Then, relax the quads, glutes, and the knee, and move the shin forward over the foot, bending the ankle, as if starting to sit on a high stool. While sinking downward, keep the spine and head in one vertical line. When the knees and ankles are bent, the pelvis is relaxed, and the back is straight, there will be a crease between the tops of the legs and the waist. Stand tall, but keep the shoulders relaxed, not lifted. Don't puff the chest. Keep the spine straight, the pelvis neutral, and the buttocks relaxed. It is not important how much the knees are bent, so long as they are bent.

When the skeleton no longer fully supports the body, we say the body is weighted. Feel the body weight going equally through each foot. Push the ground through the gushing springs point and feel how the ground pushes back.

This posture is known as the horse stance. It is one of the most fundamental of all martial arts postures. For reference, look on the internet at photos of athletic young children surfing. They are naturally in a horse stance. It is the primary posture in Pole Standing, mentioned earlier. Double-weighted sitting exercises such as the horse stance increase strength and stability. By lowering the body's center of mass and then holding this bent knee and ankle position, the postural muscles are activated to keep the body balanced.

Using a clock, hold the posture for as long as possible. That time will become the benchmark. Then hold it for longer the following day. This is a serious balance exercise with big balance benefits. Aim for 15 minutes. As the posture is held for more time, everyday balance will improve. *Figures 14, 15 & 16.*

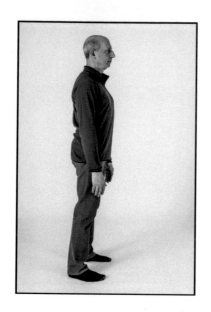 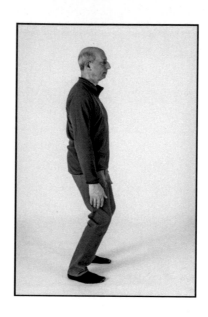 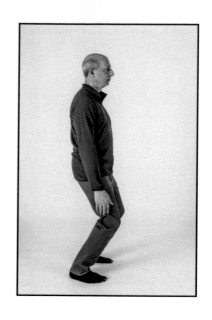

Figure 14: Feet straight, parallel, and even

Figure 15: Knees and ankles bent moderately

Figure 16: Knees and ankles bent more – compare with knee and shin in previous photo

Single-Weighted

There is more stability on one leg with bent knee and ankle and relaxed pelvis – a single-weighted posture - than on two legs, bent or straight. Surfers stay upright standing on one bent leg. Skiers shift weight from one leg to the other. Figure skaters perform powerful movements standing on the tip of one skate. T'ai Chi movements are organized around a one-leg stance.

In single-weighted Postural Retraining™ exercises, the line of gravity is an imaginary line of support where body weight goes through the gushing springs point of the standing foot. This allows a person to relax the knee and ankle and push down to increase stability, or to rotate on the ball of the foot, as in figure skating. This posture is the holy grail of standing stability. It is the template for Postural Retraining™. *Figures 17 – 36.*

Weight Transfer*

Double-Weighted to Single-Weighted

Stand with legs comfortably spread apart and slightly bent, in one of three positions: At arm's length, and at a right angle to, a wall or a support bar, just touching with the tips of the fingers of one hand. Or, face the wall at arm's length and touch the wall with the fingers of two hands. Or, stand at right angles to the wall, put hand on hip, elbow up and to the side, and just touch the wall with one elbow. The goal is to stand without support, using the wall only for balance.

50/50 (Both Feet on the Ground)

Touch the wall or bar, for balance only, with the fingers of the right hand, with both hands, or with the tip of the elbow. Slide the left or outer foot* up to touch the right or inner foot*, keeping both feet on the ground, 50/50 weight. Keep your knees relaxed and slightly bent. Then move the left foot back. Repeat ten times.

Touch the wall, for balance only, with the fingers of the left hand, with both hands, or with the tip of the elbow. Move the right or outer foot to touch the left or inner foot, keeping both feet on the ground, 50/50 weight. Keep your knees relaxed and, if you can, slightly bent. Then move the right foot back. Repeat ten times.

This exercise is practice for standing on both legs when they are equally weighted, whether they are spread apart, or close together.

0/100 (Big Toe of Outer Foot Touching the Floor)

Do the same as 50/50 above, but when the outer foot touches the inner foot, lift the heel of the outer foot until the big toe is only touching the ground for balance, with 100% of body weight on the inner foot. Keep the toe of the outer foot touching the ground for balance but bearing no body weight. Keep the knees relaxed and slightly bent. Repeat ten times on each side.

This exercise teaches how to transfer body weight from one leg to the other, while remaining balanced: in this case, from 50% on both legs to 0% on one leg and 100% on the other.

0/100 (Foot Lifted)

Do the same as 50/50 above, but when the outer foot touches the inner foot, wrap the top of the outer foot around the upper ankle/lower calf of the inner leg. The outer foot is off the ground. Keep the knee of the standing leg relaxed and slightly bent. Touch the wall or bar for balance only. Hold for as long as possible. Congratulations! This is a single-weighted stance! Repeat ten times on each side.

This exercise teaches the postural muscles to balance the body on one bent leg, just as athletes do.

Focus on these three exercises until it is comfortable to go further. The following exercises require a partner, unless falling is not an issue.

0/100 (Foot Lifted High)

Use the right-hand fingers for balance. Keep the right knee relaxed and right leg slightly bent. Do the same as 50/50 above, but when the outer foot touches the inner foot, lift the left leg until the thigh is as high as the waist, the shin is at a right angle, and the toes are pointed down. Hold up the left leg with the left arm. Repeat ten times. Turn around and switch hands and legs. Hold up each leg for as long as possible.

This exercise relaxes the back and teaches the postural muscles to balance the body on one bent leg when the other leg is raised and lowered.

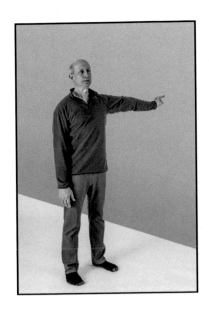 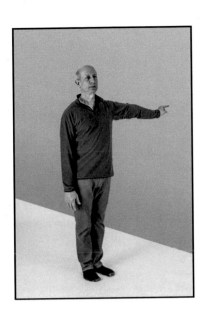 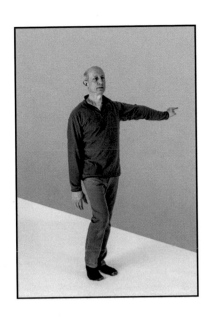

Figure 17: Touching the wall at a right angle, weight 50/50, legs apart

Figure 18: Move outer foot to inner foot, weight 50/50

Figure 19: Feet together, lift the outer leg until it has 0% weight, and 100% weight on the inside leg

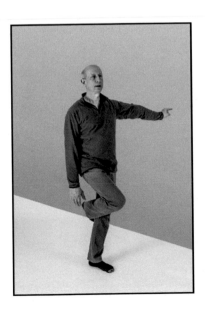 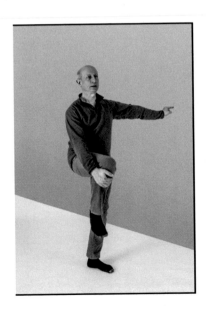

Figure 20: Foot wrapped around the calf

Figure 21: Leg raised high

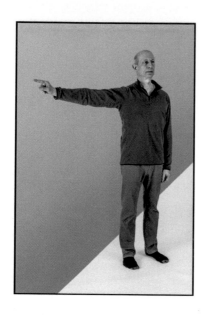

Figure 22: Switching sides

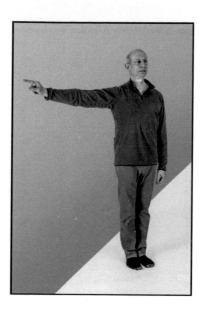

Figure 23: Move outer foot to inner foot, weight 50/50

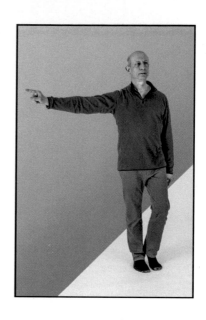

Figure 24: Weight 100% on inside leg, 0% on outer leg.

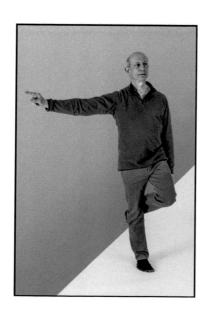

Figure 25: Foot wrapped around the calf

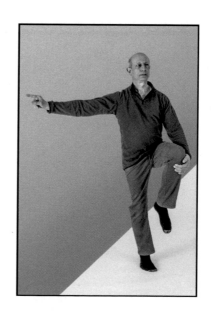

Figure 26: Leg held high

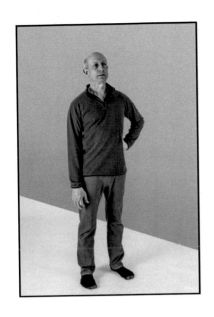

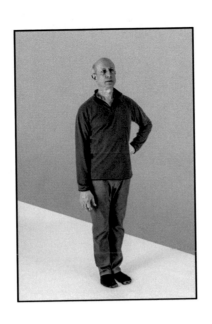

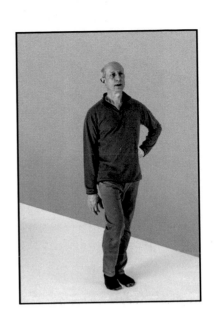

Figure 27: Touching wall with elbow

Figure 28: Move outer foot to inner foot, 50/50 weight

Figure 29: Weight 100% on inside leg

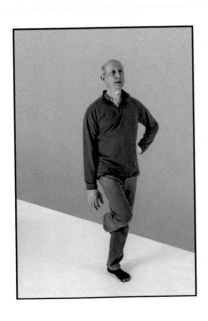

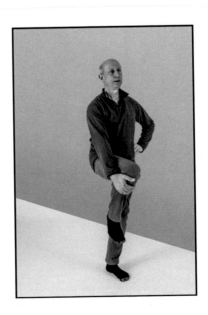

Figure 30: Leg wrapped around calf

Figure 31: Leg held high

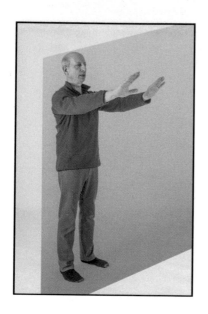

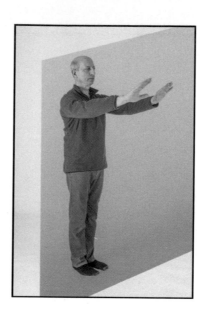

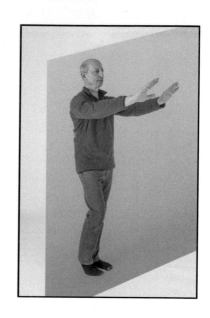

Figure 32: Facing the wall

Figure 33: Move one foot to the other, weight 50/50

Figure 34: Lift one foot onto the toe, weight 100% on other leg

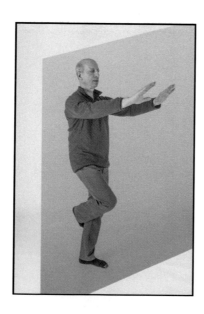

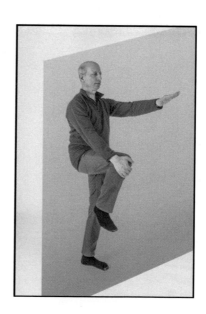

Figure 35: Foot wrapped around calf

Figure 36: Facing wall, leg raised high

0/100 Big Sidestep

Stand with knee bent and one foot lifted high at the waist, shin at a right angle, toes pointed down. Lower that foot through the body center and step one shoulder width sideways. As the foot lands, lift the other foot high. Hold the thigh as high as possible, the calf at right angles, and point the foot down. Alternate back and forth. The longer the 100% weighted leg position can be held, the better.

This exercise teaches the postural muscles to balance the body on one bent leg, while stepping sideways. *Figures 37 – 43.*

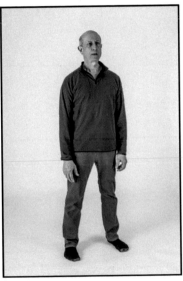

Figure 37: Weight 50/50

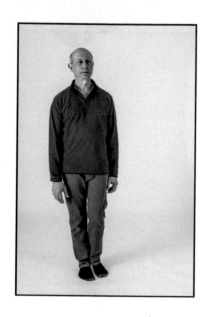

Figure 38: Weight 100% on inside leg

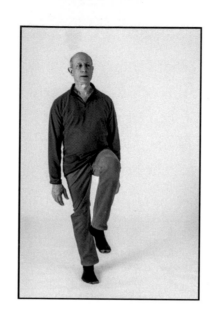

Figure 39: Lift the leg and hold

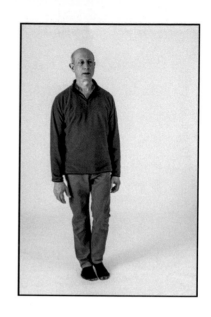

Figure 40: Lowering the leg straight down with no weight

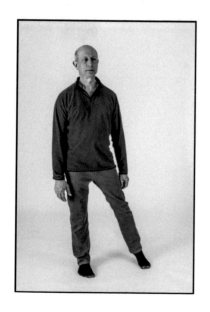

Figure 41: Move leg to the side

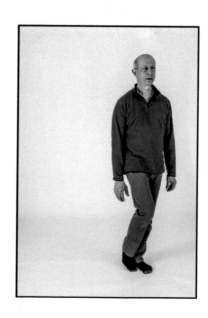

Figure 42: Weight 100% with stepping leg, move standing leg over with no weight

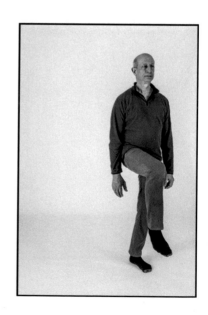

Figure 43: Raise the moving leg and hold

Forward and Back

Stand with one leg bent and forward, the other leg straight and back. Straighten the forward bent leg by sitting back and bending the back leg. Then straighten the back leg and bend the front leg. This is one cycle. Do ten times, then switch legs. The goal is to have 100% weight on the bent leg so the straight leg can be lifted and moved above the floor.

Do the same exercise, but move one foot to the other, the rear to the front, then the front to the rear.

These exercises teach the postural muscles to balance the body while moving forward or back. *Figures 44 – 58).*

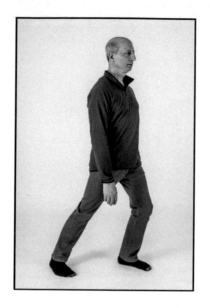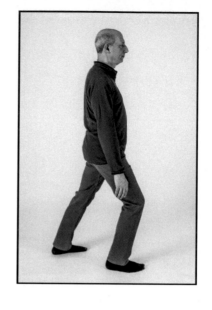

Figure 44: Weight on lead leg 70%, rear leg 30%

Figure 45: Reversing lead and rear legs

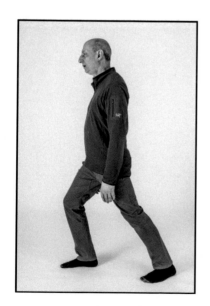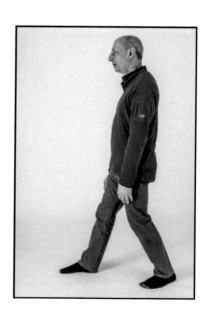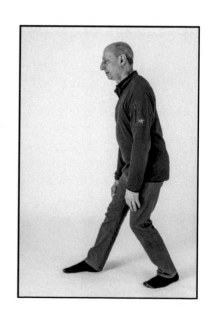

Figure 46: Weight bent lead leg 70%, rear straight leg 30%

Figure 47: Weight 100% rear bent leg, 0% weight straight front leg.

Figure 48: Bad posture. Hip tilted to the rear, back and neck not vertical.

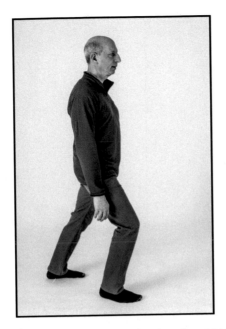

Figure 49: Weight 70% leading leg, 30% rear leg.

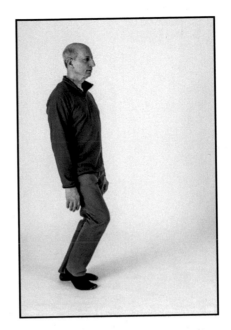

Figure 50: Bring lead leg back by placing weight 100% on rear leg

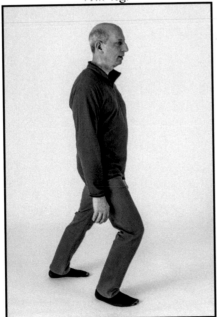

Figure 51: Step with unweighted leg so lead leg is weighted 70%

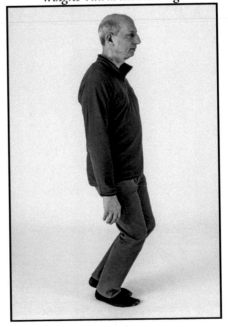

Figure 52: Bring rear leg to lead leg, weight 100% lead leg, 0% rear leg

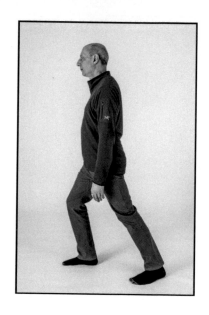

Figure 53: Weight 70% lead leg, 30% rear leg

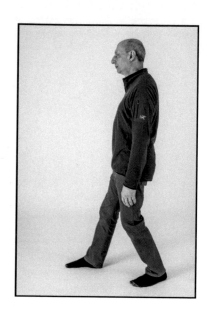

Figure 54: Weight 70% rear leg, 30% front leg

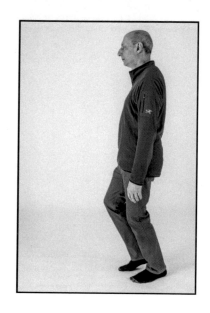

Figure 55:Rear leg weight 100%, lead leg weight 0%

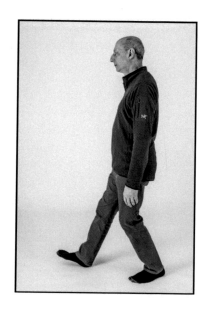

Figure 56: Step forward lead leg weighted 30%, rear leg 70%

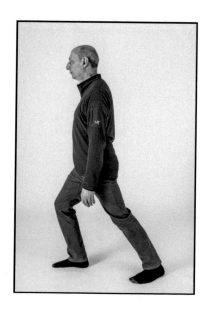

Figure 57: Continuing step, lead leg 70%, rear leg 30%

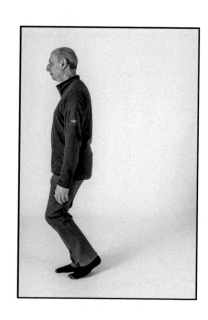

Figure 58: Lead leg weighted 100%, rear leg weighted 0%

Taking a Step

In a normal step, body weight is fully transferred from the rear foot to the lead foot* before the lead foot touches the ground. At some point, it is impossible to take the step back. Instead, become single weighted and gradually bend the knee of the weighted leg. At the same time, extend the straight and unweighted leg lightly across the floor to the front. Practice extending and retracting the lead leg. This is called making length* by lowering the body. When the extended foot is at the desired spot, slowly transfer the weight from the rear foot to the lead foot. The lead foot has time to get into a secure position, and the step can be completed or taken back.

This exercise teaches how to take a step securely and incrementally. *Figures 59 – 63.*

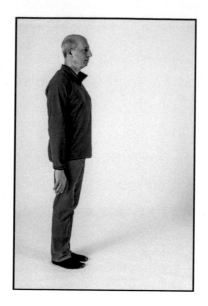

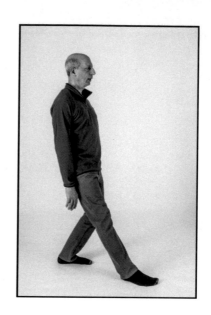

Figure 59: Stand legs together weight 50/50

Figure 60: Weight 100$ rear leg, 0% on the front leg.

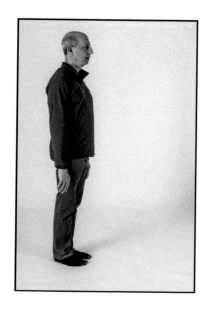

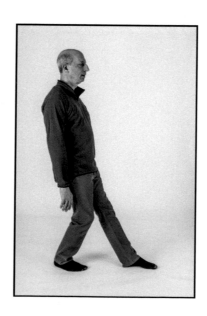

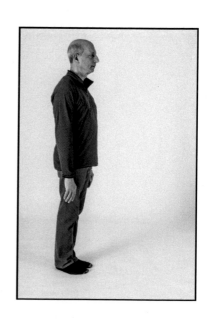

Figure 61: Move lead leg back, weight 50/50

Figure 62: Weight 100% on rear leg, lead leg 0%

Figure 63: Weighted 50/50

Turning the Body

Stand straight with legs spread, bend and put 100% weight on the left leg, extend the right leg, and turn the entire body counterclockwise as many degrees as you are able and comfortable remaining balanced on the left leg, so that the right foot reaches its place lightly and without any body weight. Do ten times on one leg, and then switch legs, weighting the right leg, and turning clockwise, moving the unweighted left leg.

No matter how much of a turn you make, always sink on the bent and weighted leg, start the turn by twisting the weighted foot, don't stand up, and extend the unweighted leg as if it's the arm of a clock. Note how sinking on the weighted leg during the turn increases stability.

This exercise teaches how to comfortably and securely turn the whole body while weighted 100% on one leg, which is a very stable way to move. *Figures 64 – 70.*

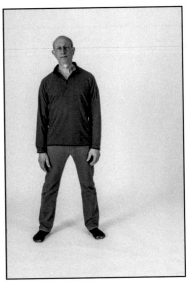

Figure 64: Weighted 50/50

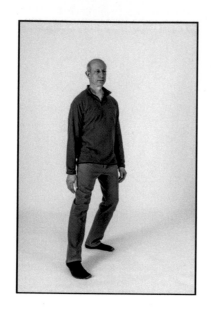

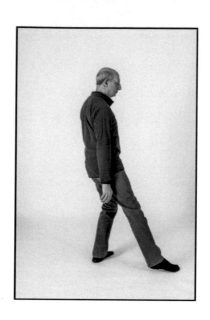

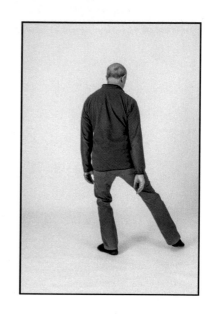

Figure 65: Weighted 100% rear leg, 0% lead leg

Figure 66: Lead leg continues weighted 0%, rear leg continues weighted 100%

Figure 67: Twist/rotate rear leg to continue turn

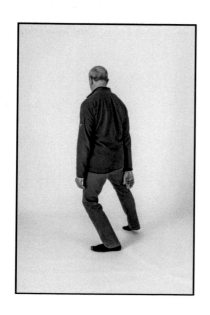

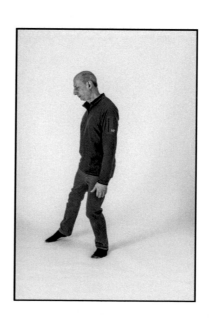

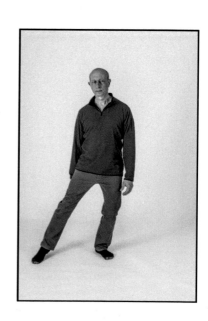

Figure 68: Lead leg still has 0% weight

Figure 69: Lead leg still has no weight, turn by twisting rear leg

Figure 70: 360-degree turn end with moving leg 0% weight.

Walking Bear

Walking Bear (name translated from the Chinese) is an exercise of weighted walking. It is an extremely stable way to move. Stand with feet touching at the heels at 45 degrees to one another. See *Figure* 12. Gradually sink on the right foot so that it bears 100% of your body weight. To do this, the right ankle is somewhat closed, the right knee is somewhat bent, the tail bone is dropped, and you are stable. This is a "sitting" position*. It is subtle not extreme.

Sit and take 100% body weight on the right, then take a step as above with the left foot at about 90 degrees to the ankle line of the right foot. Place the left foot on the ground and step. By slowly and evenly transfering 100% body weight from the right leg to the left leg and foot. Then bring the right foot, which is not carrying any weight, up to the left foot which is carrying 100% weight. *Do this all this without standing up.* Close ankles and bend knees to avoid standing up. Then turn 90 degrees and "sit" on the left foot and take 100% body weight and take a step as above with the right foot at 90 degrees to the ankle line of the left foot. Place the right foot on the ground and step. Slowly and evenly, transfer 100% body weight from the left leg to the right leg and foot. Then bring up the left foot, which is not carrying any weight, up to the right foot which is carrying 100% weight—all without standing up. This is one repetition. Do as many as possible.

This exercise teaches an extremely stable way to walk, *Figures 71 – 90.*

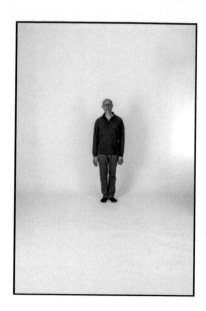

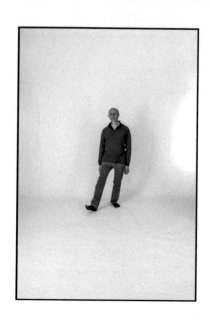

Figure 71: Weight 50/50, feet at 45-degree angle

Figure 72: Step with lead foot 45-degree angle to rear foot, lead leg 0% weighted, rear leg weighted 100%

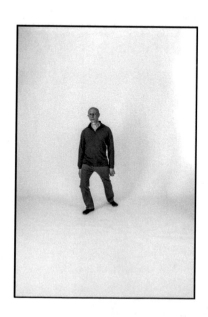

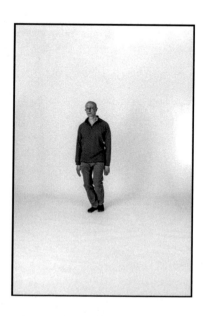

Figure 73:Step on lead leg weighted 70%

Figure 74: Lead leg weighted 100%, bring up rear leg no weight

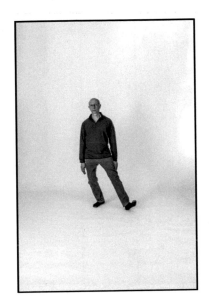 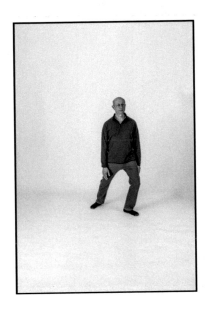

Figure 75: Rear leg becomes lead leg, no weight

Figure 76: Step with lead leg weighted 70%

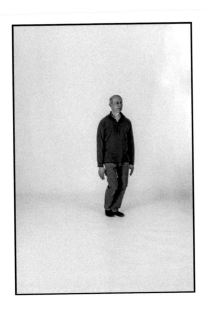

Figure 77: Lead leg 100%, rear leg comes forward with 0% weight

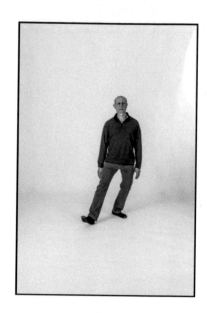

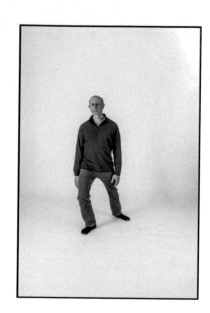

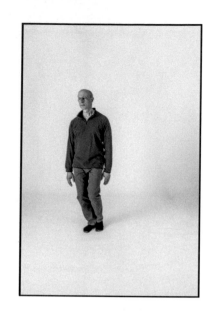

Figure 78:Rear leg becomes lead leg with no weight

Figure 79: Rear leg becomes lead leg weighted 70%

Figure 80: Bring rear leg forward with no weight, lead leg 100%

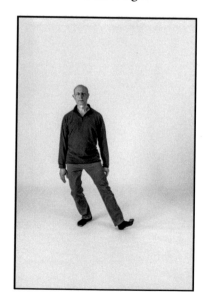

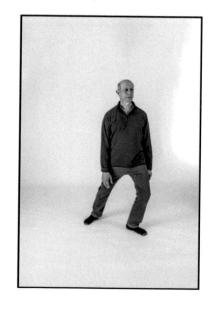

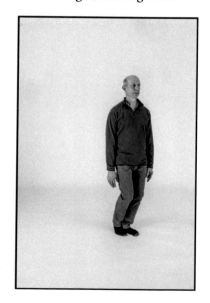

Figure 81: Step at 45 degrees, lead foot has no weight

Figure 82: Weighted 70/30

Figure 83: Bring rear leg up to front leg, keep rear leg unweighted and lead leg weighted 100%

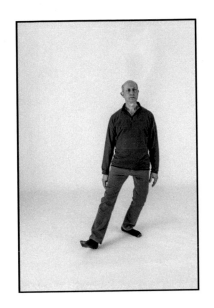

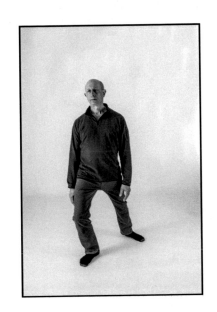

Figure 84: Lead leg steps 90 degrees from rear leg, with no weight

Figure 85: Lead leg weighted 70%, rear leg weighted 30%

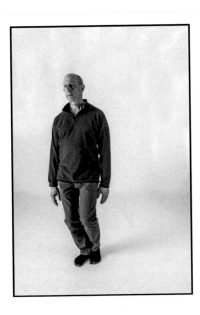

Figure 86: Bring rear leg to lead leg, rear leg weighted 0% and lead leg 100%

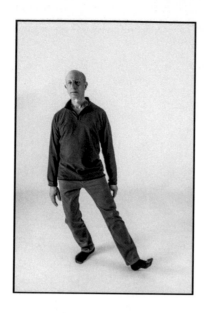

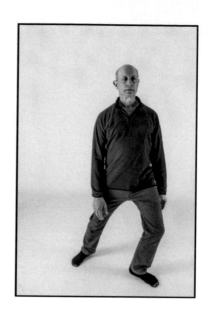

Figure 87: Lead leg steps 45 degrees from rear leg, 0% weight on lead leg

Figure 88: Lead leg 70% weight, rear leg 30% weighted

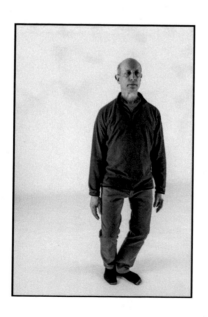

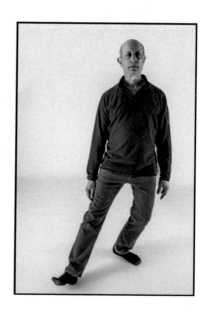

Figure 89: Bring rear leg to lead leg, rear leg 0% weight, lead leg 100%

Figure 90: And so on ...

Standing Bear

Standing Bear (name translated from the Chinese) is a deceptively difficult exercise that incorporates three principles of T'ai Chi movement: being single weighted, shifting weight between legs without standing up, and rotation of the hip (where the femur bone meets the pelvis). The Chinese call this joint the *Kwa**. It is not the waist, which is higher up.

Stand with legs spread comfortably about shoulder width apart. Put 100% body weight over the left leg. The left foot points forward, the left calf points forward, the left knee is over the toe, the tailbone is dropped, and the back is lengthened upward. Turn (close) the kwa to the left while keeping the left leg weighted. Close the kwa until the leg posture above can't be kept straight and the hip begins to turn. Then stop the turn. This is closing the kwa, not twisting the spine, and not rotating the waist or shoulders.

After completing the turn, sit back without standing and place 100% body weight over the right leg, in the same posture as for the left, and close the kwa on the right side until the leg posture above can't be kept straight, and hip begins to turn. Then stop the turn.

Keep going from one side to the other, at a slow rate of speed, for at least 15 minutes a day. *When sitting back in either direction, do not stand up. Rather, always keep the waist at an equal distance from the ground. In order to do this, bend the ankle and knee of the foot taking the weight.*

This amazing exercise facilitates the rapid and stable transfer of body weight from one leg to another, facing in either direction. *Figures 91 – 103.*

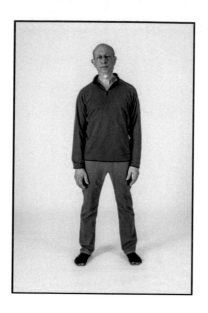

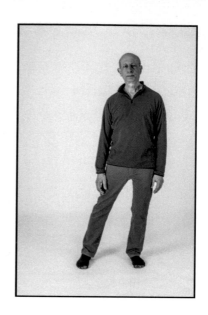

Figure 91: Stand with legs weighted equally

Figure 92: Move the body over one bent leg weighted 100% and one straight leg weighted 0%

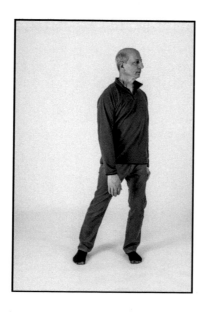

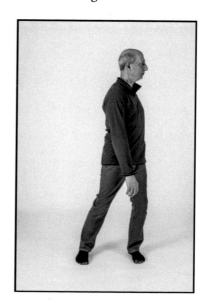

Figure 93: Turn the body to face the direction of movement. Keep weight on the bent leg!

Figure 94: Continue to turn the body and keep weight on the leg that is bent.

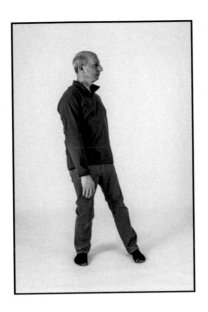

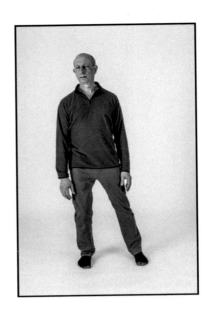

Figure 95: Straighten bent leg and without standing up move body to other leg while bending it

Figure 96: Begin to turn the body toward the bent and weighted leg

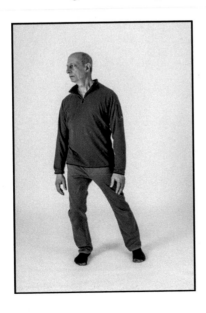

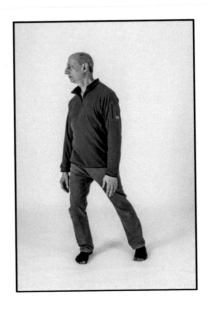

Figure 97: Continue to rotate body toward bent leg that is weighted

Figure 98: Continue to rotate the body toward the bent weighted leg

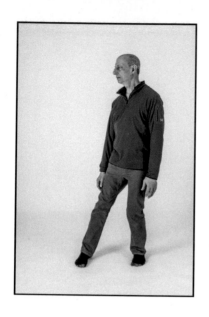

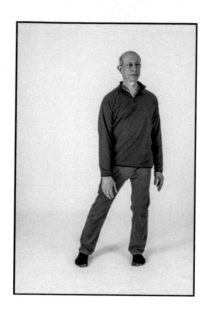

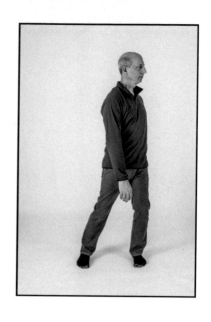

Figure 99: Straighten bent leg and without standing up shift weight to other bent leg – this is one repetition

Figure 100: Continue to rotate body to the bent leg

Figure 101: Continue to rotate toward weighted bent leg

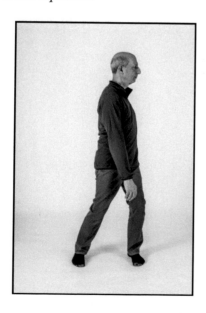

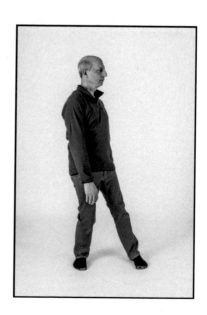

Figure 102: Complete rotation facing weighted bent leg. Note the straight and parallel feet

Figure 103: Straighten the leg without standing up while bending the other leg – continue the movement

Stretching the Tendons and Ligaments of the Arms and Hands

Stand with legs spread. Raise arms to shoulder height and extended them to either side, arms slightly bowed forward (in front of the shoulder line, not behind it), with hands pointing to the sky at 90 degrees to the arm (or as much as possible), palm and fingers open. Keeping the arms straight, stretch/push the arms outward/away from the body, leading with the top of the palm, thereby stretching the hands and the fingers. Don't puff the chest.

Notice the tightness and physical blockages* wherever they manifest. Holding this position may feel uncomfortable, but the discomfort will often disappear if the position is held. The longer the posture is held, the more the arms and hands will be stretched. It is a powerful self-massage.

This exercise is self-treatment for carpal tunnel syndrome, hand cramps, tennis elbow, and other hand/arm issues. *Figures 104 – 106.*

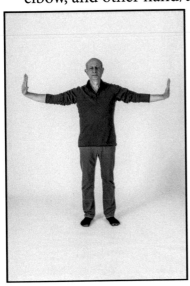 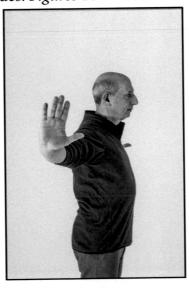 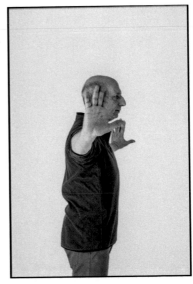

Figure 104: Arms straight but elbows not locked, hands and fingers at right angles.

Figure 105: Wrong position. Arms should be in front of shoulders, stomach and chest should be in, not puffed out.

Figure 106: This correct position will take time. The arm and hands tend to be tight and difficult to stretch.

Standing Up From a Chair

Standing from a chair is a good exercise for balance and for strength. Work with a partner. Sit in a hard chair with arms, but don't use the arms. Practice standing using only the legs. If the feet, walker, etc. are placed too far forward of the chair - what usually happens - the torso and the legs become separated. Seniors are taught to "let gravity help them to stand up" by placing their legs forward of the chair, swinging the torso forward over the legs and feet, and then standing up! In other words, to fall forward as the first part of rising.

Instead of falling forward, sit on the front edge of the chair, but pull the feet as far back as possible. Place the feet *underneath* the seat of the chair, behind the front legs of the chair. The body will be over the feet, rather than behind them, The legs can push the body straight up to standing from the *yongquan*/gushing springs point in the ball of the foot, without swinging the arms and without falling forward.

The key is to sit on the front edge of a hard chair, place both legs underneath the seat of the chair, not in front of it, and push straight up with the legs. *Figures 107 – 112.*

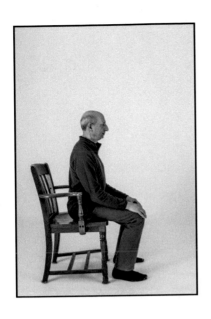

Figure 107: Feet too far forward. Very typical and very wrong.

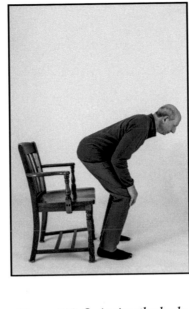

Figure 108: Swinging the body over the feet is a forward fall. Not recommended!

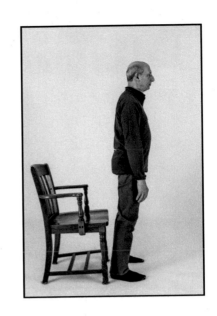

Figure 109: The idea is to stand when weight is over the foot, i.e. before falling forward on the face.

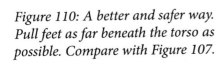

Figure 110: A better and safer way. Pull feet as far beneath the torso as possible. Compare with Figure 107.

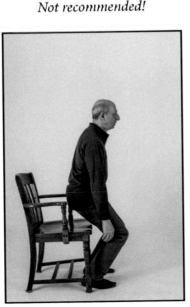

Figure 111: Push straight up from a position of balance and stability Don't swing!

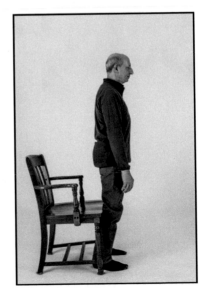

Figure 112: Feet are under the chair; the body is stable and ready to step.

Sitting Down in a Chair

Sitting in a chair is more of a challenge to balance and strength than standing up from a chair. Work with a partner. Practice with a sturdy wooden chair with arms. Stand and back up to the chair until the backs of both legs touch the chair. Look behind and place each hand as close as possible to the arms of the chair. While pressing the backs of both legs against the seat of the chair, *face forward* and begin to sit until the hands touch the arms of the chair. Do not twist in order to hold with one arm. Sit down until both hands touch the arms of the chair. If there are no arms, keep the arms at the side and feel for the seat of the chair. Then, sit down using the arms and legs for control. The key is to touch the chair with the back of the legs, and then touch with both hands, without turning around, and control the descent with the arms. *Figures 113 – 118.*

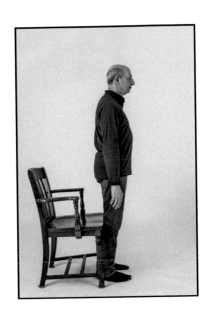

Figure 113: Stand with back of both legs touching a solid chair

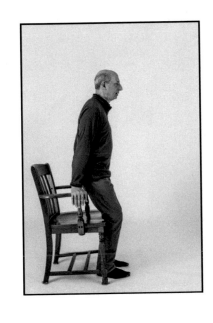

Figure 114: Put both hands on both arms of chair without looking back.

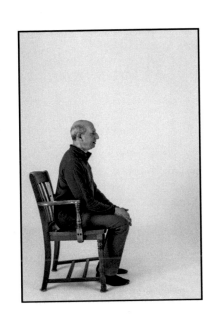

Figure 115: Seated. Note that the feet end up under the seat. See Figure 110.

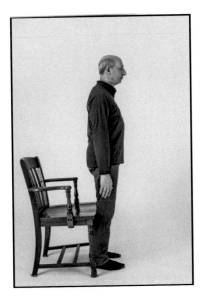

Figure 116: If the chair has no arms, feel for the seat.

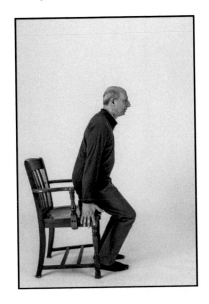

Figure 117: Don't turn around and keep both arms extended

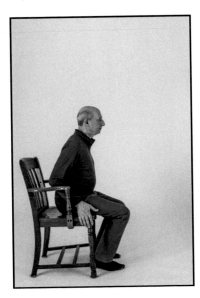

Figure 118: Only practice on a sturdy chair and with a partner.

Squatting

If there is such a thing as the best exercise in the world, it would be squatting. It is only fitting that the best is saved for last!

Squatting stretches the ankle, bends the knees, strengthens the legs, stretches and lengthens the lower back, and relaxes the pelvis. Billions of people around the world, usually in the "less-developed" countries, squat rather than stand.

Always work with a partner unless you are an athlete and able to fall without a problem. Keep the exercise area clear. If exercising alone, hold onto something solid in front, such as the leg of a heavy table. It is important to do the exercise correctly, even though the body will always search for an easier way to do it. If it is easier, it means it is incorrect.

Stand with legs close together and feet pointed forward, bend the knees and slowly lower the body as far down as possible keeping the feet flat on the floor. The neck and back are straight. Bend the knees by bringing the shin forward over the foot and lower the tail bone down toward the floor, as if sitting on a very low stool. *Take care not to fall backwards.* Stay higher, rather than sticking the buttocks back to get lower; don't drop the head or angle the torso in order to seem to go lower. Only squat to the extent that the straight back posture can be maintained while the hip is lowered. When close to the floor, wrap the arms around the legs and squeeze. Keep the heel flat on the floor, the foot pushes against the floor at the *gushing spring* point just below the ball of the foot.

Hold this position for a couple of minutes. This is a sustained posture, not a repetition exercise. Always begin the squat by moving down from standing, not by moving up from the ground. This is likely to take a few years to achieve, but so what?

In the popular western squat, as the knees bend, the top of the back is tilted forward and down toward the legs, and the buttocks is pointed back, known as the anterior tilt. Examples abound on the internet. The Postural Retraining™ squat, which is entirely different than the western squat, maintains a vertical and straight neck and back.

The long-term goal is to go from standing into the squat with feet together and pointing straight ahead (not angled outward), the neck is straight (not tilted forward), the back is vertical and straight (do not bend at the hips or arch the back), the pelvis is relaxed (in a neutral position), the tail bone is a few inches above the ground, feet are flat with weight on the balls of the feet (not the heel), and both arms are wrapped around the legs. This exercise has no performance goal other than to do it. The benefits will be enormous. *Figures 119 -122.*

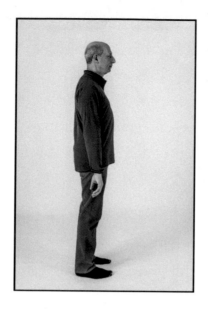

Figure 119: Begin the squat from standing

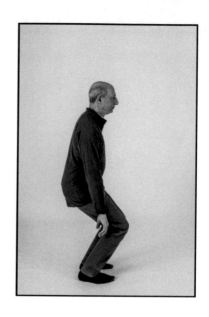

Figure 120: Sinking deeper keeping the neck and back straight and pelvis relaxed. To go beyond this point, the legs must be strong.

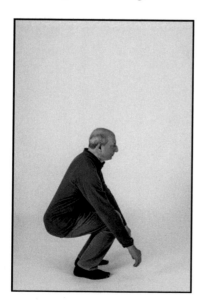

Figure 121: To go beyond this point, the lower back and ankles must be loose

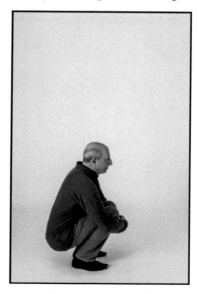

Figure 122: Body weight through the balls of the foot, pelvis relaxed and a few inches off the floor, back and neck straight, squeezing the shins toward the torso.

Pain

Because Postural Retraining exercises are sustained, and the knees and ankles are bent, it is likely that the legs will ache, or even shake. Muscle aches and shakes are natural. If able, continue the exercise even if uncomfortable, because this builds capacity, which leads to fewer aches and pains. Self-monitoring is important. In the event of sharp ongoing joint pain, stop that exercise and do another. Try again the next day. Or do a different exercise. Don't stop altogether!

Patience

The Chinese word for patience translates as "open heart." Postural Retraining™ is not easy, but it is not that difficult. Have a good attitude and an open heart because these exercises will be a new experience. It takes time and effort to relearn balance. Practice Postural Retraining™ with the diligence and commitment of an infant learning to stand.

Reward

Ahh! The balance you lost has returned! What reward could be greater? Congratulations! Keep it up and spread the word!

AFTERWORD

///

Further Research

Researchers and organizations interested in evaluating Postural Retraining™ as a fall prevention program, using experimental or quasi-experimental design, or for peer review[18] should contact the author at glocker@mindspring.com.

Is Postural Retraining™ T'ai Chi?

Postural Retraining™ draws deeply from the well of T'ai Chi wisdom and my teachers. It is derived from and inspired by T'ai Chi, but it is not T'ai Chi. T'ai Chi is not an exercise for the elderly in which you move slowly and wave your arms. That is called dancing, and T'ai Chi is not dancing.

T'ai Chi Chuan—the more modern English spelling is *Taijiquan*—translates from the Chinese as "Great Ultimate Fist" (*Chuan* being fist). It is an advanced and physically challenging martial art, one of any number of fighting "chuans." T'ai Chi is practiced for a lifetime, and it takes decades to achieve some level of mastery. At 82, Master Yu's martial skills were astounding.

In China, a study of T'ai Chi would be undertaken after years of basic martial arts exercises involving fast punching and kicking forms. My T'ai Chi form is comprised of 108 postures; the transitions between the movements are single weighted with bent knees and ankles; and it takes 45 minutes to complete. It is not easy.

Medical doctors now routinely recommend T'ai Chi to their older patients. That advice comes at least 30 years too late. So-called elder T'ai Chi and its many spin-offs

---

18 https://www.ncoa.org/center-for-healthy-aging/basics-of-evidence-based-programs/apply-ebp/falls-prevention-programs/

rarely if ever incorporate the bent knee and ankle and weighted posture of the real thing. Elder T'ai Chi is not conceived or presented as a challenging weighted exercise. Quite the opposite. Consequently, the benefit to postural muscle balance is minimal.

Seniors rightly find the hand movements in elder T'ai Chi to be complicated, puzzling, and too much to memorize. While it is true that doing something that resembles T'ai Chi is certainly better than doing nothing[19], elder T'ai Chi is not challenging enough.

Postural Retraining™ exercises are more beneficial than elder T'ai Chi because they are true weight-bearing exercises, which stimulate the postural muscles to bring the body into balance.

Finally, if Postural Retraining™ is inspiring, join a serious mixed-age T'ai Chi class.

---

19 https://www.nytimes.com/2018/09/10/well/move/using-tai-chi-to-build-strength.html

GLOSSARY OF TERMS*

//

6   Exercise – Where body weight is transferred from one leg to the other and the torso moves.

6   Posture – The body is held still in a certain position and the legs do not move. Also known as an "at rest" or "static" position or posture.

11   Quadriceps (quads) – The major muscles of the front of the thigh.

11   Gluteus (glutes) – The major muscles of the hip.

12   Weight-bearing exercises – Bending the knees and ankles while keeping the head and back straight and sustaining the posture. This activates the postural muscles to balance the body. Because the postural muscles are held at a constant length, and the angle of the joints does not change, standing with bent knee and ankle is a whole-body isometric exercise. It is the heart of Postural Retraining™.

16   Gravity – One of the forces of nature by which all things with mass are brought toward one another. On earth, gravity gives weight to physical objects.

16   Volitional muscles – The phasic or action muscles, which are controlled by conscious thought, intent, and direction. The mind can direct a leg to lift.

16   Weightlifting exercise – Repeated contraction of a muscle under resistance, which changes the size of the muscle and the angle of the joints. Also known as an isotonic exercise.

17   Non-volitional muscles – The postural or balance muscles, which are not subject to conscious direction. The mind cannot direct a leg to balance.

18   Weighted – Where the leg or legs support the mass/weight of the body, and the percent supported, from 0 to 100. By leaning the body, bending the knee and ankle, or lifting a leg, a person who weighs 150 lbs. can support 150 lbs. on one leg (single-weighted), support 75 lbs. on each of two legs (double-weighted equally), or support 150 lbs. In an uneven split, 30% (45 lbs.)/70% (105 lbs.) (double-weighted unequally).

18   Weight-bearing sport – Incorporates a posture where the knees and ankles are bent and held that way for a sustained period. Examples include surfing and skiing.

19   Dropping body weight – When the body is slightly lowered by bending the knees and ankles, while keeping the head and back straight. Can be done standing on one or two legs. Also known as "sitting." If done quickly and then arrested at the foot, considerable downward force can be created, which is stabilizing.

20   Balance – Using the postural muscles to stand erect and upright with no destabilizing force other than gravity.

20   Stability – When faced with a destabilizing force in addition to gravity, using the postural muscles, and generating downward force in excess of mass, to remain upright.

21   Ground Reaction Force – The reaction of the ground equal to the downward force exerted against it, but in the opposite direction. The existence of the two forces results in an enhanced connection between the foot and the ground, which is independent of the size of the base of support.

21   Downward Force – The force going into the ground through a person; typically, their weight. Downward force in excess of body weight can be developed by rapidly closing the ankle, and lowering the knee and the center of mass, by correctly leveraging, torqueing, and rotating the joints, or by using isometric muscle action and breathing, all to increase the force in the foot pushing into the ground.

21   Newton's Third Law – For every action, there is an equal and opposite reaction. Example: A person at rest standing on the ground who weighs 150 lbs. exerts a downward force of 150 lbs. The ground exerts 150 lbs. of force toward the person in the opposite direction, known as the ground reaction force. Any increase in downward force leads immediately to an equal increase in the ground reaction force in the opposite direction. The downward force and the ground reaction force do not cancel one another out because each force is acting on a different object (the body acts on the ground and the ground acts on the body). Where and to what degree the ground reaction force moves within the body is a question waiting to be researched.

21   Newton's Second Law – Force = Mass x Acceleration (F=MA). Although a person's mass is constant, rapid downward acceleration and torqueing can increase downward force beyond body weight to enhance stability.

21   Center of Mass – An imaginary point within the body and below the navel around which the weight of the body is equally distributed. Sometimes called center of gravity.

22   Frictional force – The horizontal component of the ground reaction force. Frictional force keeps the foot from sliding on the floor, a key component of stability.

22   Rooting – An enhancement of the connective forces between a person and the ground by increasing downward force, which increases ground reaction force and frictional force.

23   Base of Support – The base of support, which is a misnomer, is defined as the area around the outside edge of the animate or inanimate object in contact with the ground, such as the feet. Widening the base of support by spreading the legs is commonly recommended for balance and stability. Postural Retraining™ does not subscribe to this point of view.

31   Moving the shin forward – if the glutes and quadriceps are relaxed, and the knee is moved downward, the shin will naturally angle toward the front of the foot.

32   Closing the ankle – When standing, bend the ankle joint by moving the knee downward causing the shin to tilt to the front of the foot. This move requires relaxation, not muscle contraction. It permits considerable dorsiflexion of the ankle. Closing the ankle lowers the body. The squatting exercise develops the ability to close the ankle

32   Bending the knee – Relax the glutes and quadriceps and move the knee in a downward direction, which will move the shin forward over the foot and bend the ankle. Note that bending the knee is entirely about being able to relax, not to flex.

32   Opening the ankle – When standing, a closed or dorsiflexed ankle is opened by moving the shin from the front of the foot to the rear of the foot, as if moving from 11 o'clock to 12 o'clock. Also known as flexion of the ankle. Opening the ankle raises the body.

35   Line of Gravity/Line of Force – The imaginary vertical line that travels through the body's center of gravity and into the ground. It represents the location and downward direction in which gravity and any other external force are acting on a person.

39   Weight transfer – In an exercise, increasing or decreasing the amount of body weight supported by one leg. Example: Going from 50/50 weight-bearing on both legs to 100% weight-bearing on one leg and 0% weight on the other.

39   Outer foot/inner foot - In a posture or exercise, the outer foot moves to the inner foot.

51   Lead foot/rear foot – In a posture or exercise, the foot in front of the torso is the lead foot, and the foot behind the torso is the rear foot.

51   Making length – To take a step by first weighting the rear leg 100% and slightly lowering the body. The lead leg can easily be extended forward of the body (i.e. lengthened) because it is not supporting any body weight. For this reason, the lead leg can be retracted, or the step can be taken.

56 Sitting - When the body is slightly lowered by bending the knees and ankles, while keeping the neck and back vertical and straight. Can be done standing on one or two legs. Also known as "dropping body weight." If done quickly and then arrested, considerable downward force can be created, which is stabilizing.

61 Kwa – Chinese name for the joint where the femur inserts into the pelvis, below the waist. It includes the iliopsoas muscle group, the adductor muscles, and the largest group of lymph nodes in the body.[20] To close the kwa means to rotate one thigh inward while holding the other thigh stationary. To open the kwa means to rotate one closed thigh outward while holding the other thigh stationary. The kwa is opened and closed independent of the waist or the shoulders. See Standing Bear exercise.

65 Physical blockages – When the torso or limb could stretch further but for tight muscles, ligaments, and tendons, which inhibit or restrict movement. Sustaining the posture, particularly when it is not comfortable, will incrementally relax and resolve such blockages.

New York, NY

February 3, 2020

20 Frantzis, *Opening the Energy Gates of Your Body,* Energy Arts Inc., Fairfax, Ca., 2006, page 163

ENDNOTES

///

Mid-Lifers: Begin Postural Retraining™ now to prevent balance and stability issues later.

Athletes: No matter how young, strong, or athletic, anyone whose sport or profession depends on standing and moving balance will benefit from Postural Retraining™. It will amplify and focus what you already have.